SAVING YOUR HEART

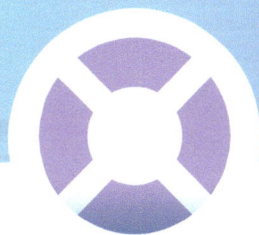

CORONARY ARTERY DISEASE AND HOW TO MANAGE IT

Coronary artery disease (CAD) is the number one cause of death in both men and women in the US. It occurs more often when you have high levels of cholesterol in your blood, use tobacco or e-cigarettes, have diabetes or high blood pressure and/or a family history of heart disease.

If you have CAD or any of the risk factors for getting it, this book can help. To prevent CAD, or to manage it, you need to know:

- what it is

- what causes it

- the signs and symptoms

- the risk factors

- what you can do

No one likes the idea of having to "manage" a disease. BUT... the fact is, if you don't manage your health, it can get worse.

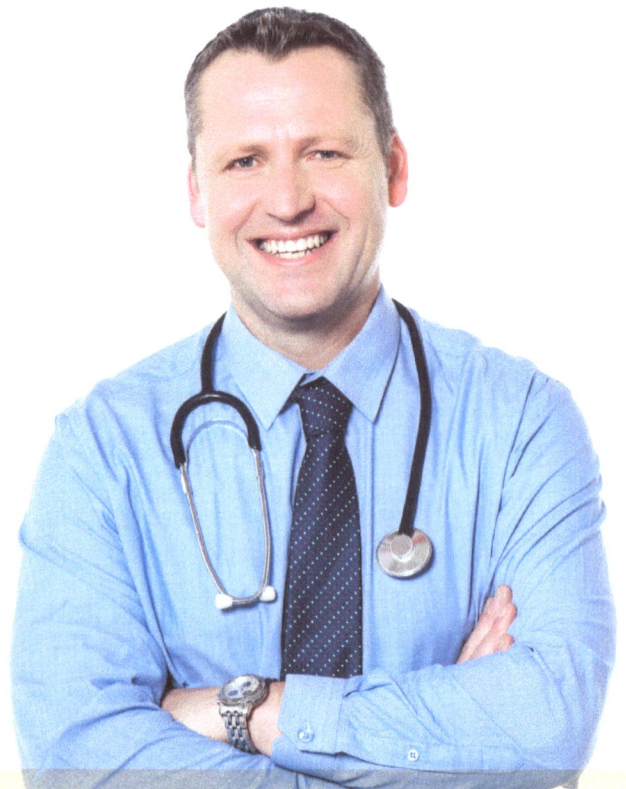

This book is to help you understand what CAD is and what you can do about it. It is only to help you learn more about CAD. It is not meant as a substitute for your doctor's advice and treatment.

The food line to your heart

The coronary arteries are the blood vessels that carry blood, oxygen and other nutrients to your heart. These small arteries are located on the outside surface of your heart muscle.

The heart needs a steady supply of blood, oxygen and other nutrients to work as it should. Over time these arteries can become clogged or blocked by cholesterol and fat deposits (called plaque). When this happens, they narrow and do not let enough blood get through to your heart.

This is coronary artery disease or CAD*.

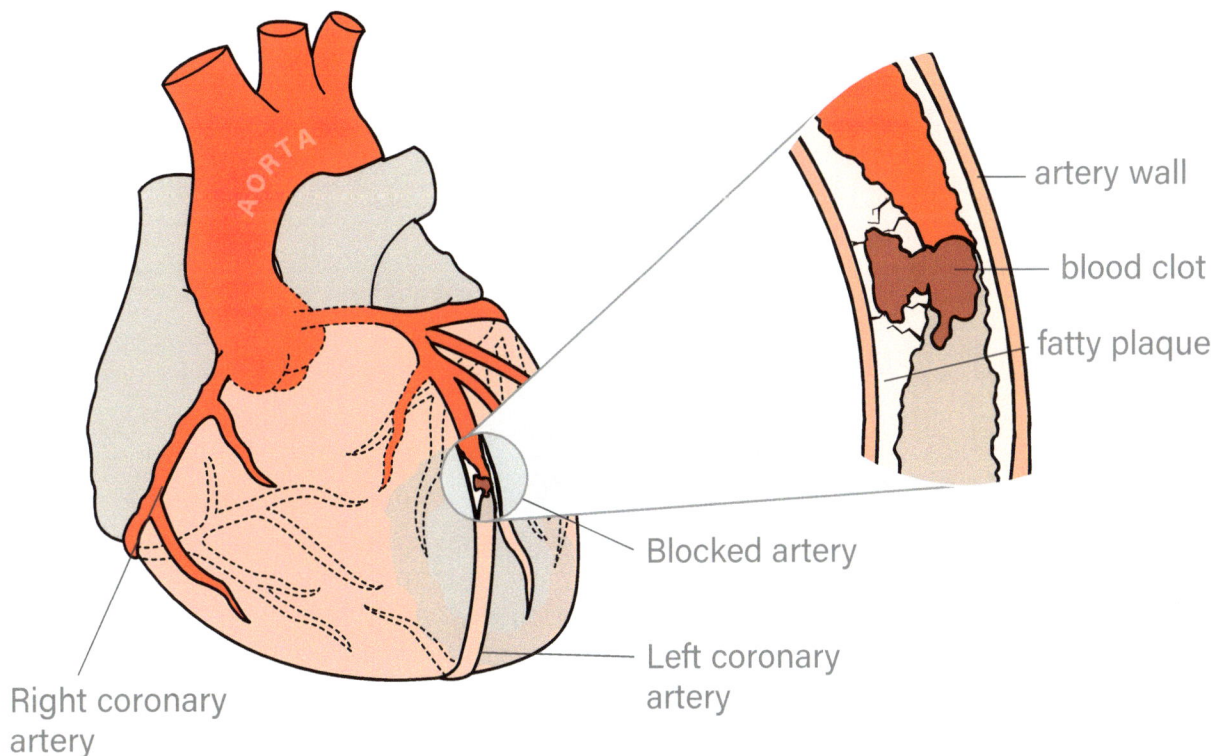

AORTA

artery wall

blood clot

fatty plaque

Blocked artery

Left coronary artery

Right coronary artery

* It is also called atherosclerosis, hardening of the arteries, CHD (coronary heart disease) or cardiovascular disease.

The cholesterol connection

Your body makes cholesterol. It is a waxy, fat-like substance that occurs naturally in the blood. It helps carry fats through your blood vessels. You also get it in some foods.

Your body uses cholesterol to help with normal body functions. However, when there is too much of it in your blood, it can cause plaque to form inside your blood vessels.

Your blood cholesterol level is made up of a variety of blood fats which include:

- LDL (low density lipoprotein)

- HDL (high density lipoprotein) and

- triglycerides (a form of fat)

Lipoproteins are complex molecules made up of fats (lipids) and proteins. Cholesterol attaches to proteins in your blood and moves along as these lipoproteins.

HDL

LDL

triglycerides

LDL cholesterol is nicknamed "bad cholesterol" because it tends to build up in arteries as plaque. When this happens, your blood vessels become narrowed and don't allow as much blood and oxygen to get through.

HDL cholesterol is nicknamed "good cholesterol" because it picks up some of the LDL as it passes through your blood vessels and removes it. But, if the amount of LDL is too high, the HDL cannot get all of them and your blood vessels start to clog.

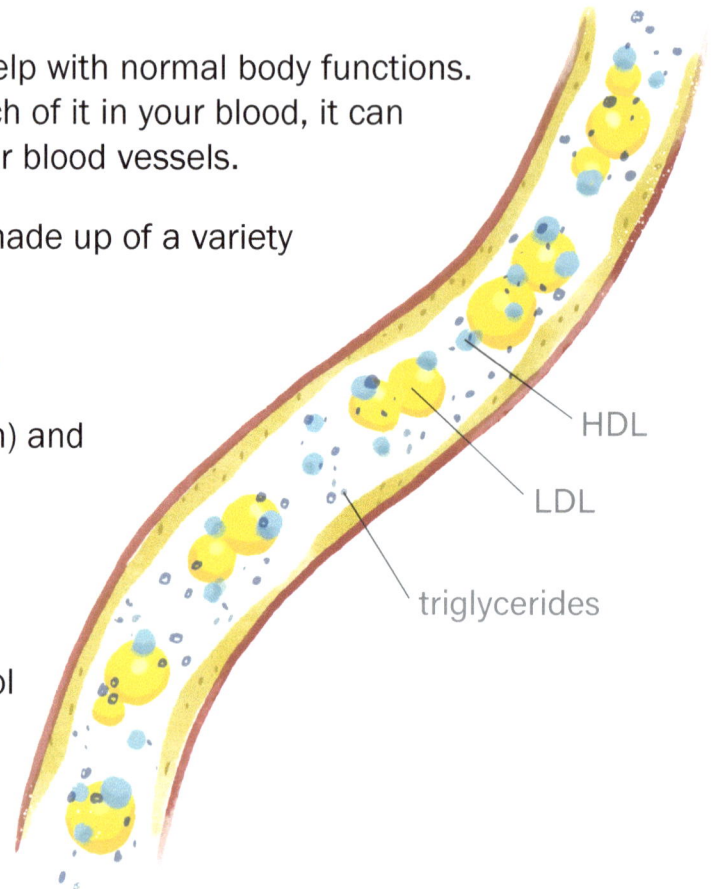

Assess your risk

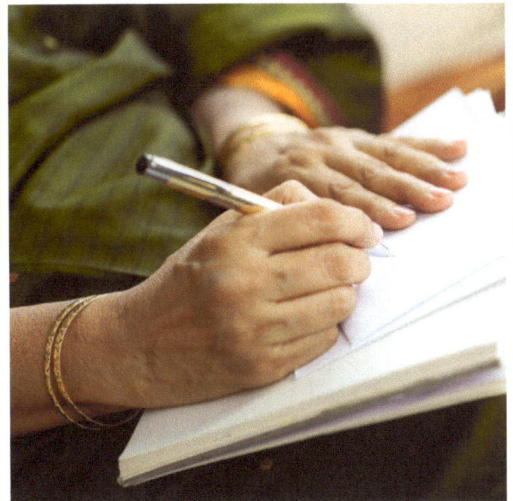

Because high levels of cholesterol in your blood lead to CAD, there are recommended levels* for adults over age 20.

Lipid blood tests	Goals in coronary artery disease or diabetes	My test results ✏️	My blood lipid goals ✏️
Total cholesterol	Less than 200 mg/dL	_____mg/dL	
Bad cholesterol (LDL)	Less than 100 mg/dL*	_____mg/dL	
Good cholesterol (HDL)	40 mg/dL or more (men) 50 mg/dL or more (women)	_____mg/dL	
Non-HDL cholesterol	Less than 130 mg/dL*	_____mg/dL	
Triglycerides	150 mg/dL or less	_____mg/dL	

* If you are at high risk for heart attack, your goal may be an LDL less than 70 mg/dL and a non-HDL less than 100 mg/dL.

The only way to know your cholesterol levels is with a blood test. Talk with you doctor about what your cholesterol levels should be—based on your risk factors, including your family history. Everyone is unique and your doctor treats YOU.

How will I know if I have CAD?

You may not have signs of high cholesterol until CAD has developed. If there is a lack of blood flow through your coronary arteries, it may begin to show up as one or more of these:

- no symptoms
- angina
- heart attack
- unusual symptoms

No symptoms

Some people with coronary artery disease may have no symptoms. They may not have any chest pain, discomfort or other signs of angina or a heart attack. Others have symptoms which are not typical. If you are not sure if your symptoms are something to be concerned about, don't wait, check with your doctor.

Without any symptoms, the disease can go along unchecked. So, learn your cholesterol levels and other risk factors in case you are one of those at risk.

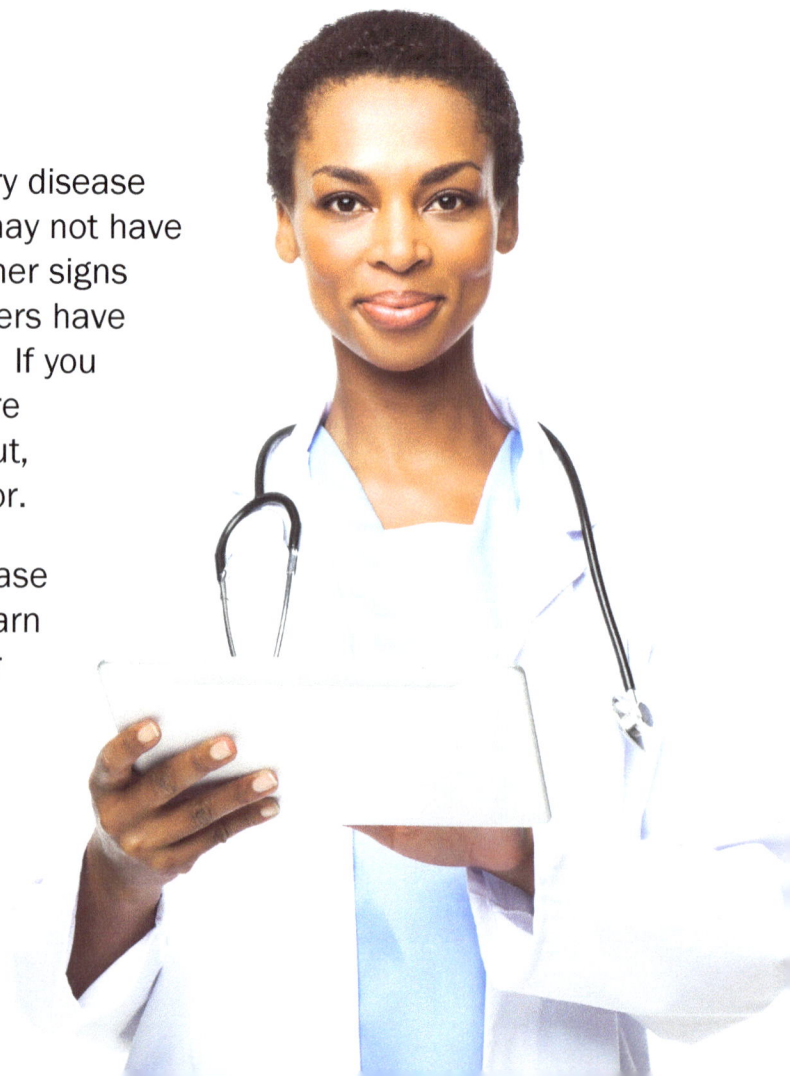

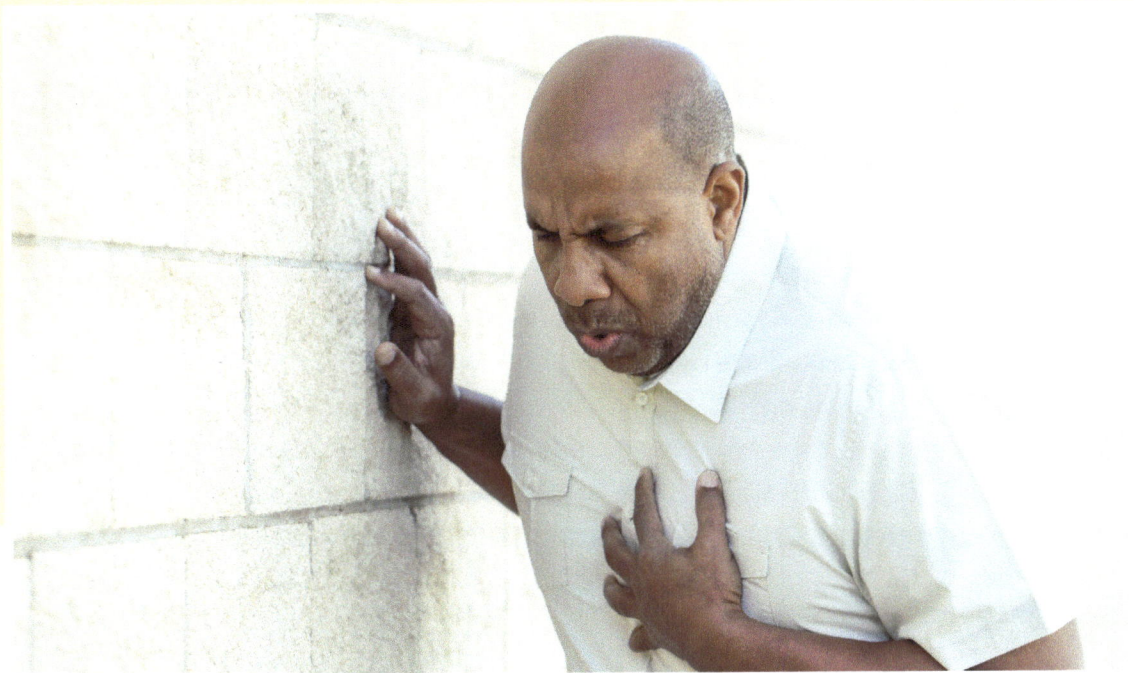

Angina

If the blood supply to your heart is cut off for a short time, your heart tissue can be damaged by the lack of oxygen.

In most cases this causes angina—the main symptom of CAD. Angina is chest pain that can feel mild, moderate or extreme. What does angina feel like?

- feels like a dull, heavy pressure on your chest

- a pain that goes out to your neck, jaw, left or right shoulder, arm or back

- a mild burning in your chest (like heartburn)

It can cause:

- shortness of breath

- fatigue (being very tired)

- palpitations (fluttery or irregular heartbeats that you can feel) instead of pain

Heart attack

Angina that does not clear up on its own or after taking medicine and lasts for over 15 minutes is most likely the sign of a heart attack.

When the oxygen supply to the heart is totally blocked in a coronary artery, heart cells die. Often, this happens when a blood clot forms. This seals off the artery and no blood can get through. The lack of blood flow causes a heart attack.

The pain felt from a heart attack varies from person to person. Any of the symptoms of angina as well as these may occur:

- sweating, "clammy" feeling skin

- skin feels cool or cold

- a feeling of indigestion or heartburn

- sharp, burning or cramping pain that starts in or spreads to the the chest, neck, jaw, throat, shoulder, upper back, arms or wrists

- extreme fatigue after activity

- nausea or vomiting

- dizziness, feeling light-headed

- shortness of breath

NOTE

Your body cannot create new heart cells after they die from lack of blood and oxygen.

Women, elderly people and diabetics often do not have "classic" heart attack symptoms. They may have less intense symptoms and more nausea.

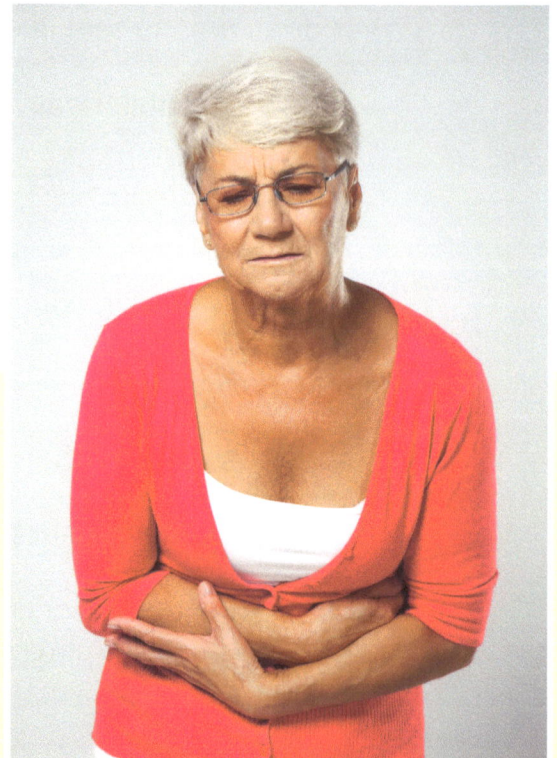

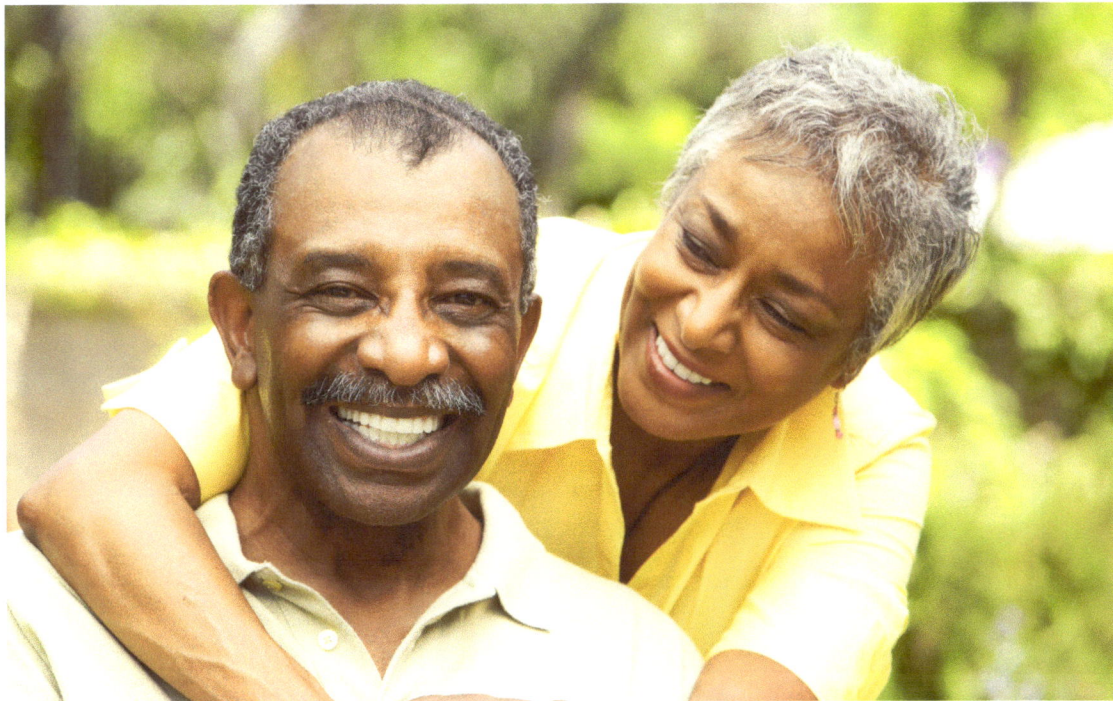

The difference between men and women

Some think that men are the only ones who need to worry about CAD. However, around the same number of women and men die each year from heart disease. And nearly two-thirds of women who die suddenly from heart disease had no warning symptoms. Women also have second heart attacks more often than men.

The difference is not whether women or men are more likely to get heart disease, but when they get it. As a rule, it takes women about 10 years longer to be at the same risk for heart disease than it does men. Natural estrogen may help protect women from the risk before menopause. After menopause, however, the gap narrows.

A woman's symptoms of CAD may not be typical, making it harder to diagnose. And, other problems may cause symptoms similar to heart disease.   For these reasons it is not uncommon for heart disease to go undetected in women.

It's risky business

Risk factors are things that add to your chance(s) of getting a disease. Some of these things can be controlled, some cannot.

There is not much you can do about:

- A family history of early heart disease. Early heart disease means:

  – your father or a brother had heart disease before age 55

  – your mother or a sister had it before age 65

- Your age. You are at risk for CAD if you are:

  – a male over the age of 45

  – a female over the age of 55

However, the majority of risk factors for coronary artery disease are not the result of aging and family history.

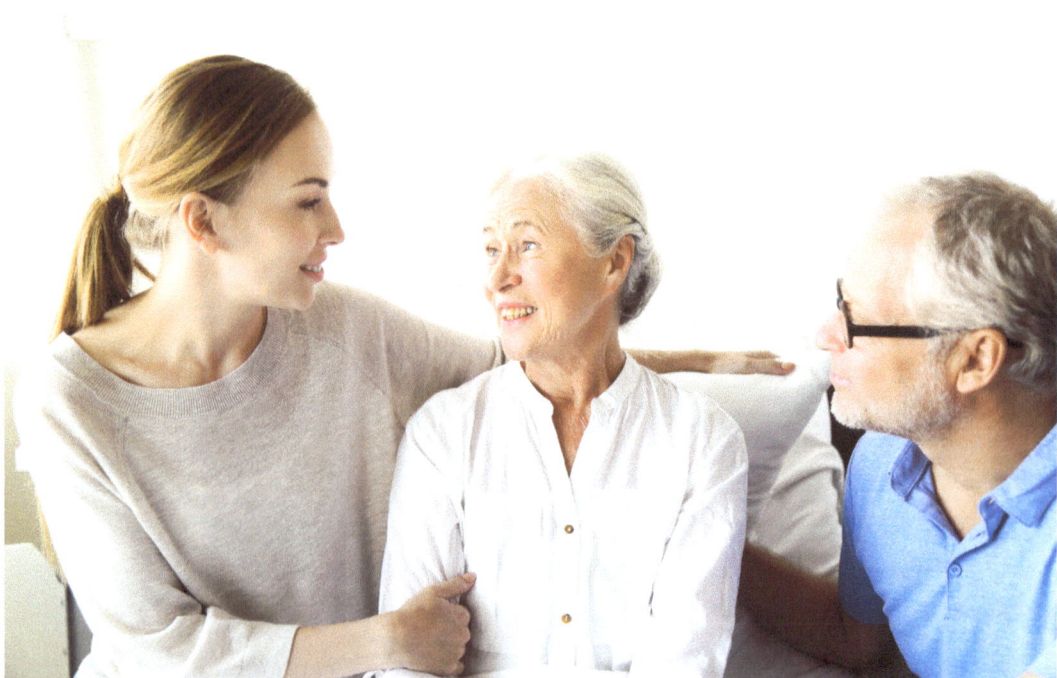

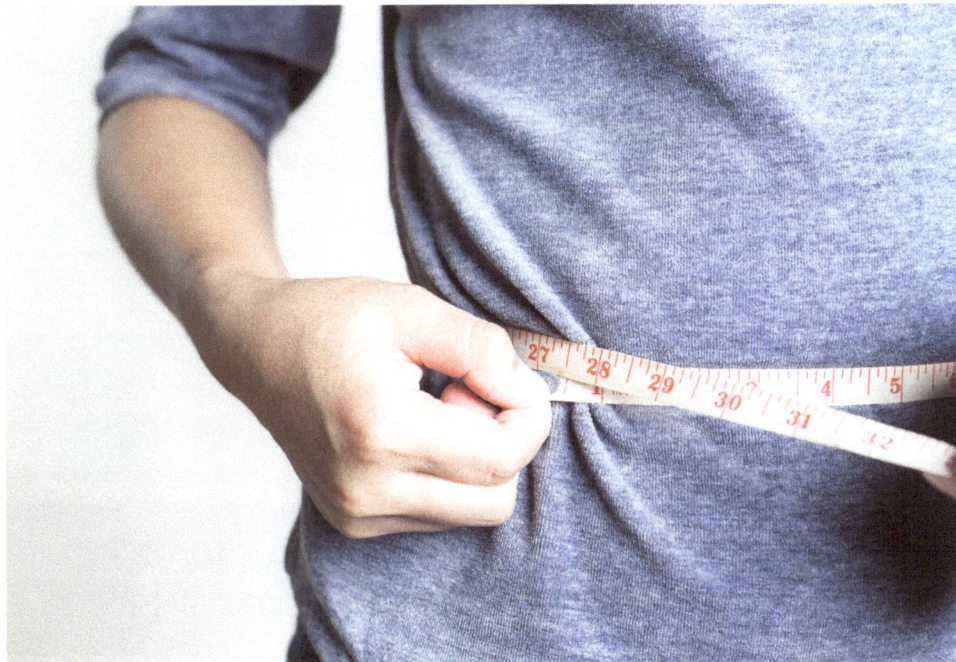

Many risk factors are related to your lifestyle, background and environment. These are risk factors you may have some control over:

- **Being overweight.** Obesity is related to high blood pressure, diabetes, high cholesterol levels and lack of exercise. All of these can lead to heart disease.

- **Having high blood cholesterol** (total cholesterol over 200 mg/dl and LDL ("bad") cholesterol over 100 mg/dl.). This is the main cause of CAD.

- **Having low HDL** ("good") **cholesterol levels** (below 40 mg/dL for men or below 50 mg/dL for women). Having HDL levels higher than 60 can offer some protection from getting heart disease.

- **Not being physically active.** Being inactive leads to being overweight, having less muscle tone and strength (including a weaker heart) and a lower HDL level. Regular, aerobic exercise helps lower your risk for heart disease. Ask your doctor what kind of exercises are best for you.

High cholesterol levels, high blood pressure and obesity often start in childhood.

- **Having high blood pressure** (higher than 140/90). When your blood pressure is high for a long time, your heart and other organs can be damaged.

- **Having diabetes.** People with diabetes have 2 to 4 times more risk of heart disease.

- **Smoking or being around others who are smoking.** Nicotine in any form damages the heart and narrows the arteries. This includes e-cigarettes.

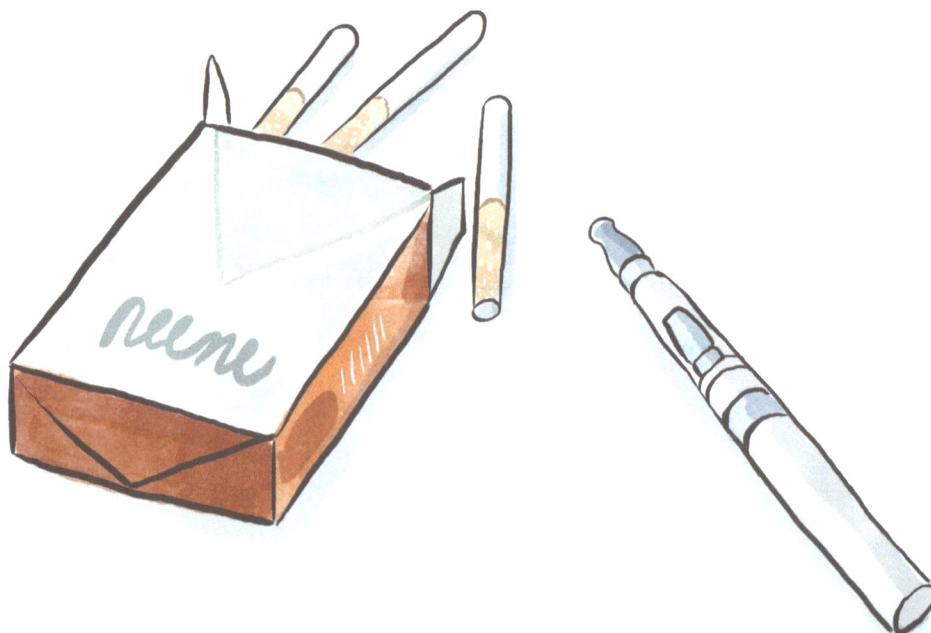

Begin today

Begin today to learn more about your risk factors. Then learn how to control the one's you can. You'll have the answer to "What can I do?"

I need to:

☐ keep my diabetes under control (see pages 14–15)

☐ stop smoking (see page 16)

☐ control my high blood pressure (hypertension) (see page 17)

☐ reduce my total blood cholesterol (see pages 18-22)

☐ reduce my bad cholesterol (LDL) (see pages 18-22)

☐ increase my good cholesterol (HDL) (see pages 18-22)

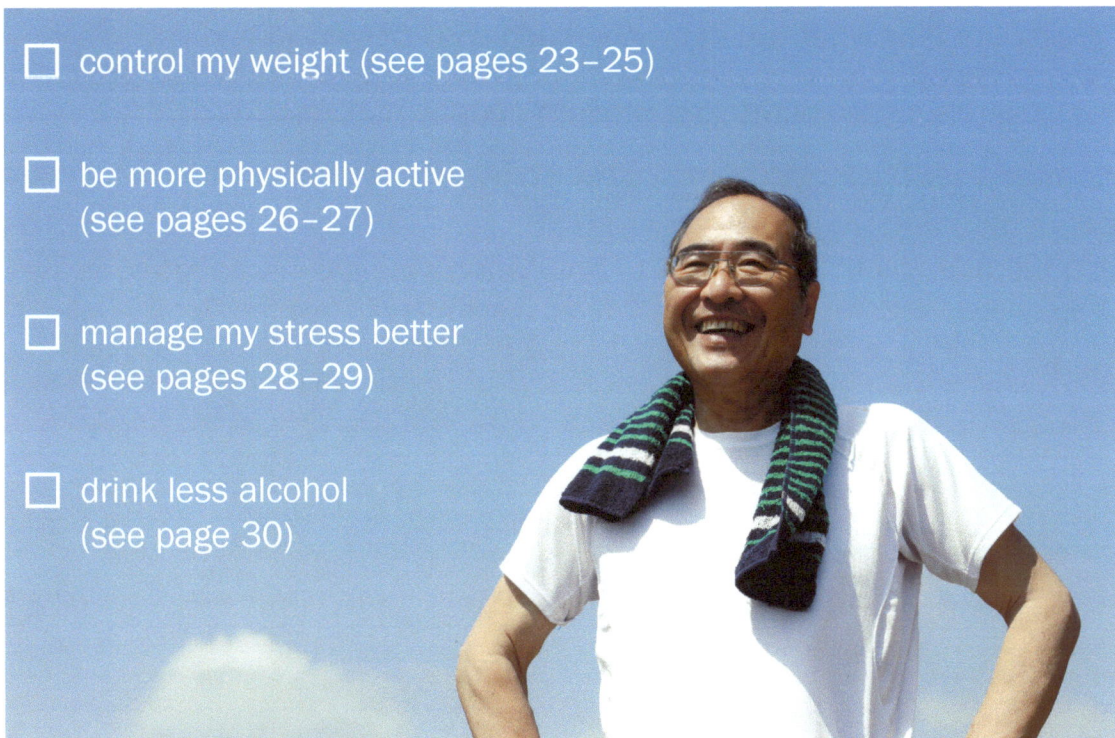

☐ control my weight (see pages 23–25)

☐ be more physically active (see pages 26–27)

☐ manage my stress better (see pages 28–29)

☐ drink less alcohol (see page 30)

Diabetes

Diabetes happens when the pancreas (an organ in your body) does not make enough insulin or your body cannot use the insulin it does make. If diabetes runs in your family, talk to your doctor about this disease. When you have a family history of diabetes it is even more important to maintain a healthy weight and exercise regularly.

If you have diabetes, you are 2 to 4 times more likely to develop CAD than someone who does not have it. This is due, in part, to insulin resistance, high blood pressure and obesity.

Diabetes increases the levels of cholesterol and fat (triglycerides) in your blood. As a result, more than 80% of people with diabetes die from some form of CAD. You also need to be aware that a person who has diabetes may not have chest pain during a heart attack.

So if you have diabetes, it is important for you to manage it. This means:

- keeping your blood glucose (sugar) within your target range

- controlling what you eat, how much you eat and when

- exercising as your doctor recommends

- keeping your weight in a healthy range

Use the diary on the next page to help you manage your diabetes.

My healthy blood glucose range is:

before meals: _____ to _____

2 hours after meals: _____ to _____

at bedtime: _____ to _____

Diabetes diary

Date	Meal Plan						Exercise	Breakfast	Lunch	Dinner	Bedtime	Medicines* (dose___)	(dose___)	(dose___)	(dose___)	(dose___)	Notes
	Breakfast	Lunch	Dinner	Snack 1	Snack 2	Exercise											

Meal Plan

Followed meal plan = 0
Varied plan a little = 1
Varied plan a lot = 2

Exercise

No exercise = 0
Light exercise (20 min or less) = 1
Moderate exercise (20-45 min) = 2
Heavy exercise (45+ min) = 3

*Medicines

Write in exact dosage taken and the time. Include herbs and vitamins.

Blood Glucose

Write in blood glucose level before meal and 2 hours after

Notes

Include signs of problems, medication reactions, how meals or activities varied from planned, etc.

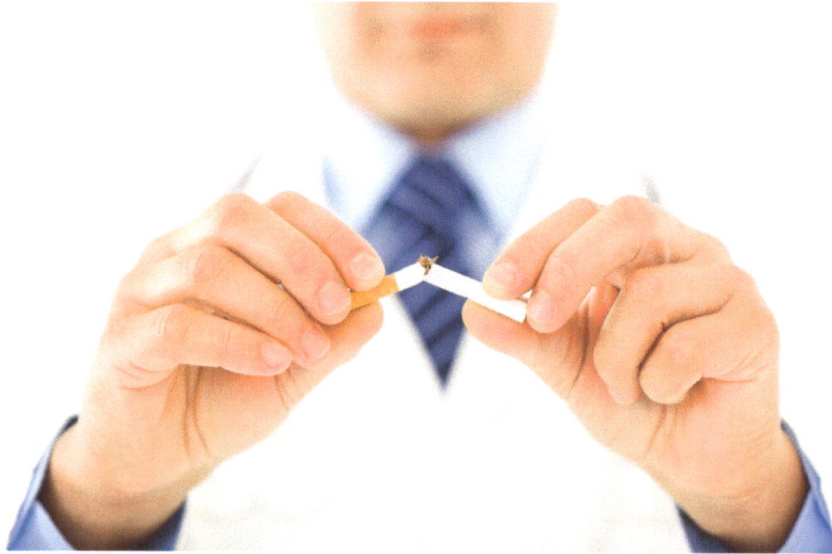

Smoking

Tobacco smoke (yours or someone else's):

- lowers your good cholesterol (HDL)

- narrows your blood vessels

- can cause artery spasms

- damages your lungs and reduces oxygen your body needs

- increases your heart rate

- shortens your life span

- adds other risks not related to your heart

Smokers are 2 to 6 times more likely to have a heart attack than nonsmokers. And, smokers who have a heart attack are more likely to die within the first hour than nonsmokers.

When you quit smoking your risk for heart disease decreases over time.

So, if you smoke, quit. If you don't smoke, don't start.

High blood pressure

High blood pressure is sneaky. You can have it and not know it. You usually don't feel a thing while it damages your arteries by letting fat and cholesterol build up. Over time, a lot of damage can be done, causing CAD or a heart attack.

High blood pressure tends to run in families and increases with age. When you have high blood pressure, at first your heart thickens. But over time it stretches and weakens. This is because the heart has to work so much harder due to the high pressure.

The good news is blood pressure can be controlled. Here's how:

- lose weight if you need to

- reduce the sodium in your diet

- exercise regularly

- take your high blood pressure medicine

- reduce your stress and relax

- don't smoke

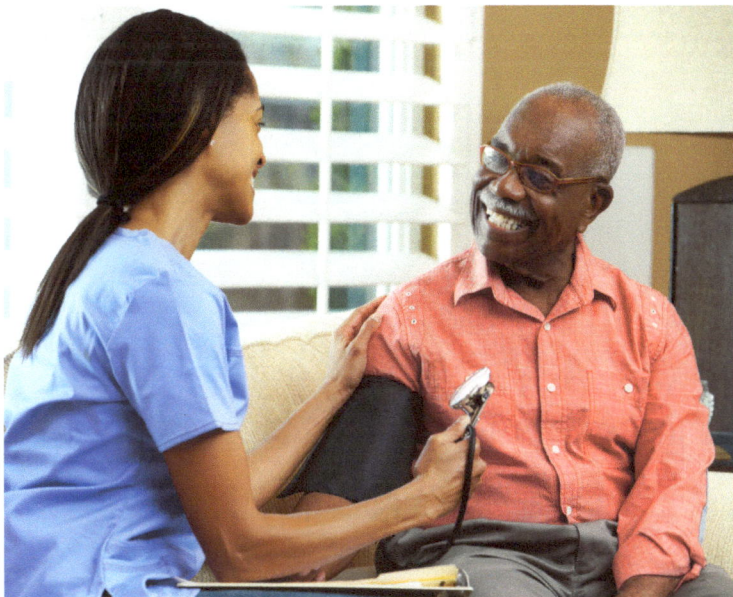

NOTE

African Americans seem to have high blood pressure more than other Americans

A high sodium (salt) diet seems to make high blood pressure worse.

Having high cholesterol

The main cause of CAD is having high blood cholesterol levels. When your cholesterol levels are high (see page 5) and you have other risk factors, you are at higher risk for developing CAD.

If you have high blood cholesterol levels, here's what you need to do to reduce these levels:

- eat a low-fat, low-cholesterol diet

- increase your physical activity

- lose weight if you are overweight

- stop smoking

- take cholesterol-lowering drugs if you need to (talk to your doctor about the benefits and possible side-effects of these drugs)

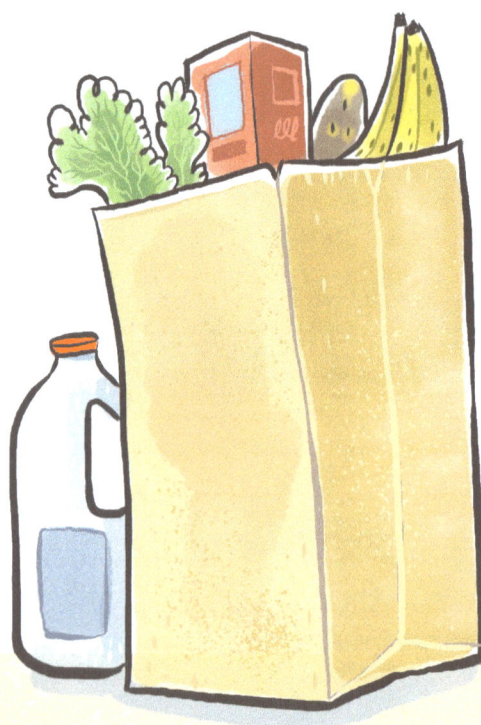

Your current cholesterol levels and whether you already have CAD will determine how much your doctor will attempt to lower your level. Talk with your doctor about what you need to do.

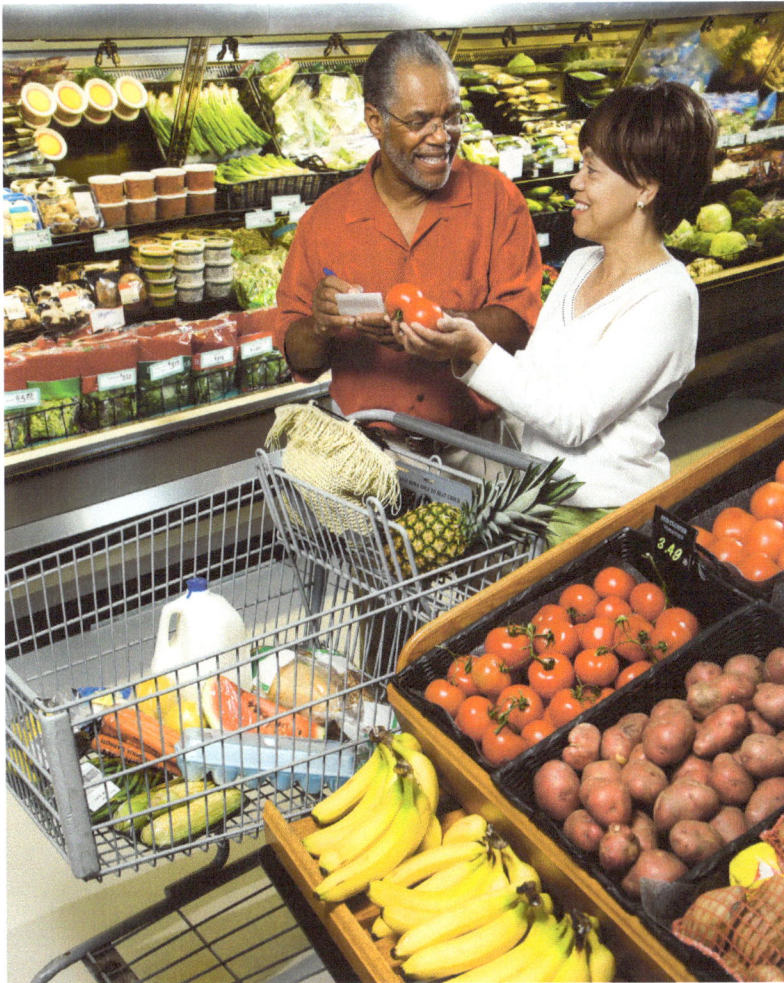

A change of diet may do wonders

Changing your diet, controlling your weight and increasing your physical activity are the first steps in treating high blood cholesterol. The first goal is to reduce bad cholesterol levels. But this goal is not a temporary "diet"— it is a permanent change in the way you eat.

Start by eating less saturated fats and high cholesterol foods. Saturated fat foods mainly come from animals. But some also come from plants (like coconut oil, palm oil or cocoa butter).

Eat more fresh fruits and vegetables. These contain very little, if any, cholesterol or fat. But be careful how you cook them or what you add to them. For example, a baked potato has no cholesterol. But if you add butter and sour cream, you've added a lot of cholesterol and saturated fat.

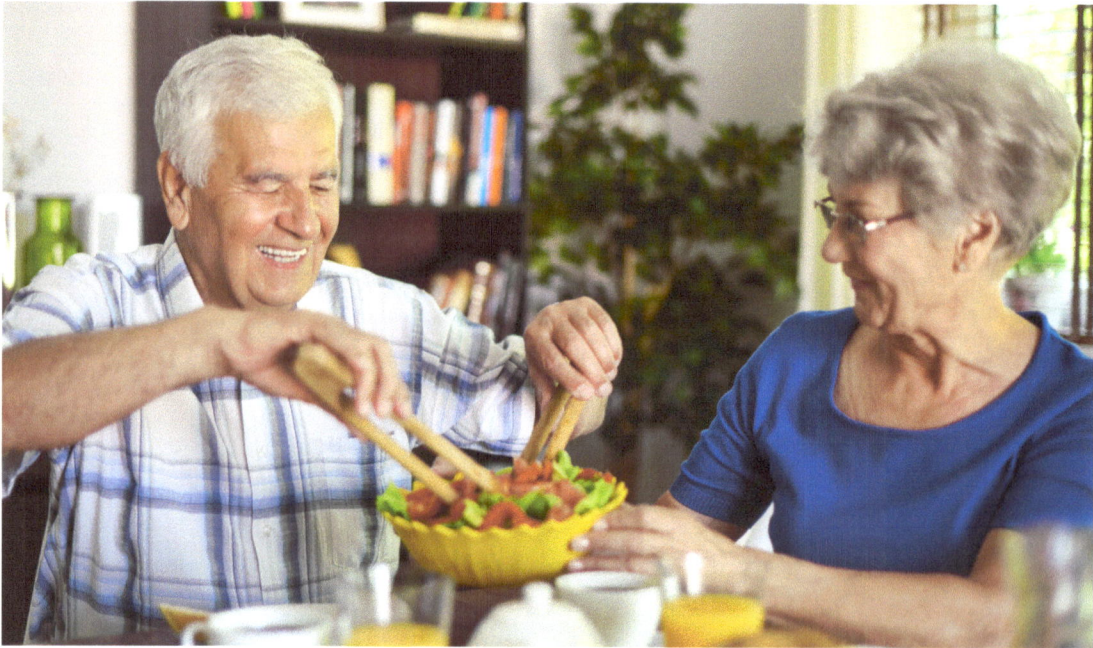

The TLC diet (Therapeutic Lifestyle Changes diet*)

The TLC diet is a healthy way of eating for the whole family. It is a low saturated fat, low cholesterol diet for your calorie needs. If you follow it, it can help in reducing your total blood cholesterol as well as your LDL cholesterol levels.

You should eat:

- less than 7% of your daily calories in saturated fat, 10% in polyunsaturated fat and less than 20% in monounsaturated fat

- 25%–35% or less of your daily calories in all fats (saturated and unsaturated)

- less than 200 mg (milligrams) of cholesterol each day

- between 50%–60% of your daily calories in carbohydrates

- between 20–30 grams of fiber each day

- about 15% of your daily calories in proteins

- enough calories to get to or keep a healthy weight (Ask your healthcare provider how many calories you need.)

* From the Third Adult Treatment Panel (ATPIII), National Institute of Health

Food labels

Watching the amount and type of foods you eat is important in trying to reduce your cholesterol levels and controlling your weight. Learn to read food labels and keep up with the amount of fat, saturated fat, cholesterol and salt you eat each day.

Most food labels list the serving size and contents (for 1 serving) of that product. The percent of daily value is based on eating 2000 calories a day. Ask your health care provider how many calories you should have each day. If you need to eat other than 2000 calories, learn how to adjust the label for your calorie needs*.

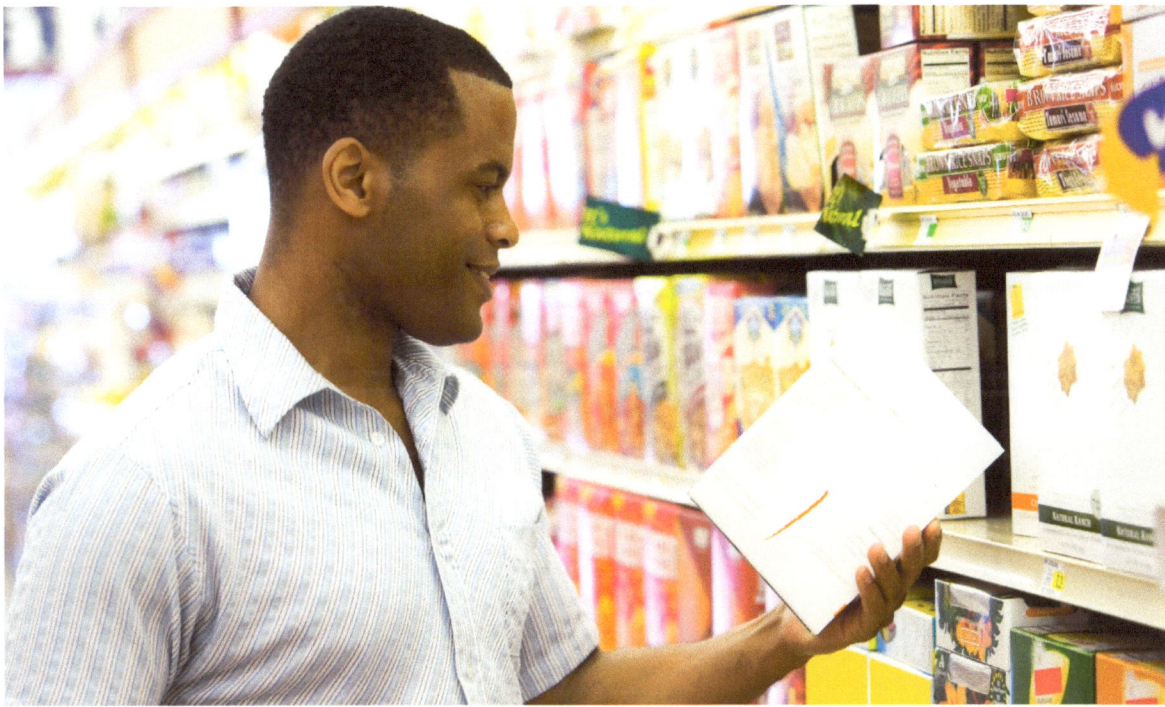

* The worksheet on the next page can help you do this. Please discuss with your doctor.

My daily diet worksheet

The number of daily calories I need are _____

Nutrient	My Daily Calories		Amount I should have	
Total Fat	_____ x .30	= _____	÷ 9 =	_____ g
Saturated Fat	_____ x .07	= _____	÷ 9 =	_____ g
Polyunsaturated Fat	_____ x .10	= _____	÷ 9 =	_____ g
Monounsaturated Fat	_____ x .20	= _____	÷ 9 =	_____ g
Carbohydrates	_____ x .50	= _____	÷ 4 =	_____ g
Protein	_____ x .15	= _____	÷ 4 =	_____ g
Cholesterol -			200 mg or less	
Sodium -			aim for 1,500 mg	
Fiber -			20 to 30 g	
Vitamin A -			5,000 IUs	
Vitamin C -			60 mg	
Calcium -			1,000 mg	
Iron -			18 mg	

Note: Keep in mind, this is not exact, but a way of keeping the food you eat in line with your needs.

The FDA and the USDA websites can give you the food label information about items that are not pre-packaged. These include fresh vegetables, fruits, meats, poultry and seafood items. Packages too small to have a label should give you an address or phone number to get the information. Make it your business to find out about the foods you like to eat.

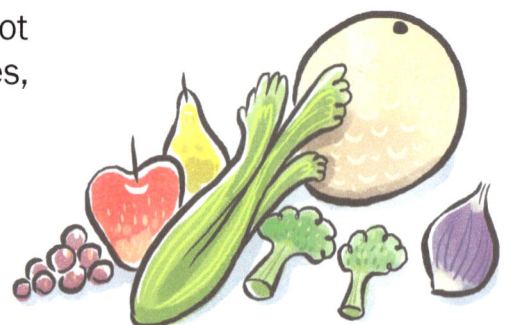

Being overweight

As your body weight increases, so does your risk of high blood pressure. You already know having high blood pressure is a risk factor for heart disease. So, keeping your weight in a healthy range is important to lowering your blood pressure and reducing your risk of CAD.

The most long-lasting and best way to lose weight is slowly. To do this, you need to use up more calories than you eat. If you cut back on your calorie intake by 500 calories a day and do some exercising, you can lose about 1 pound a week. That's 52 pounds in a year! Cut out 500 snack calories a day and see what happens.

It's not just the type of food you eat that's important. It's also the amount of food you eat. Take smaller helpings of high calorie, high fat foods. Take larger helpings of foods that are high in fiber because fiber tends to make you feel full so you eat less.

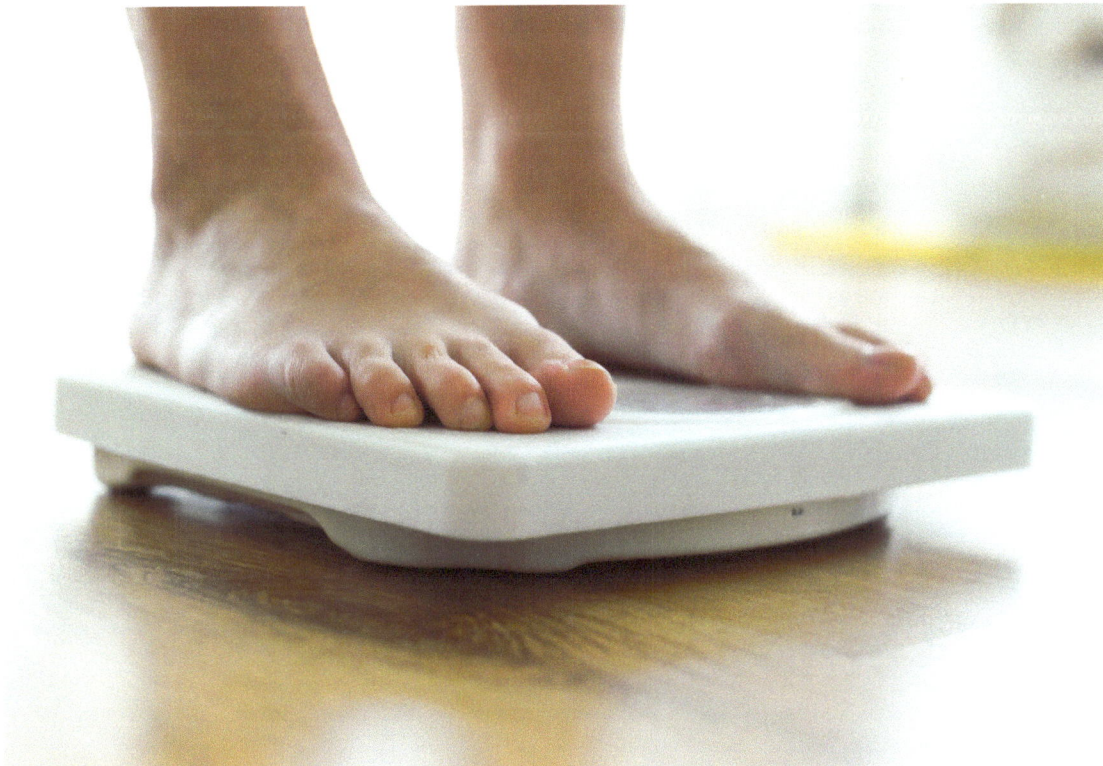

Losing weight and keeping it off may mean a new way of eating, and adding exercise to your life. Here's how to eat healthy and get on your way to a lower weight:

- Choose foods low in calories and saturated fat.

- Choose foods high in fiber.

- Limit your serving sizes.

- Become more active.

- Cut back on snacks. If you do snack, make it fresh fruit, vegetables or air-popped popcorn (without salt or butter).

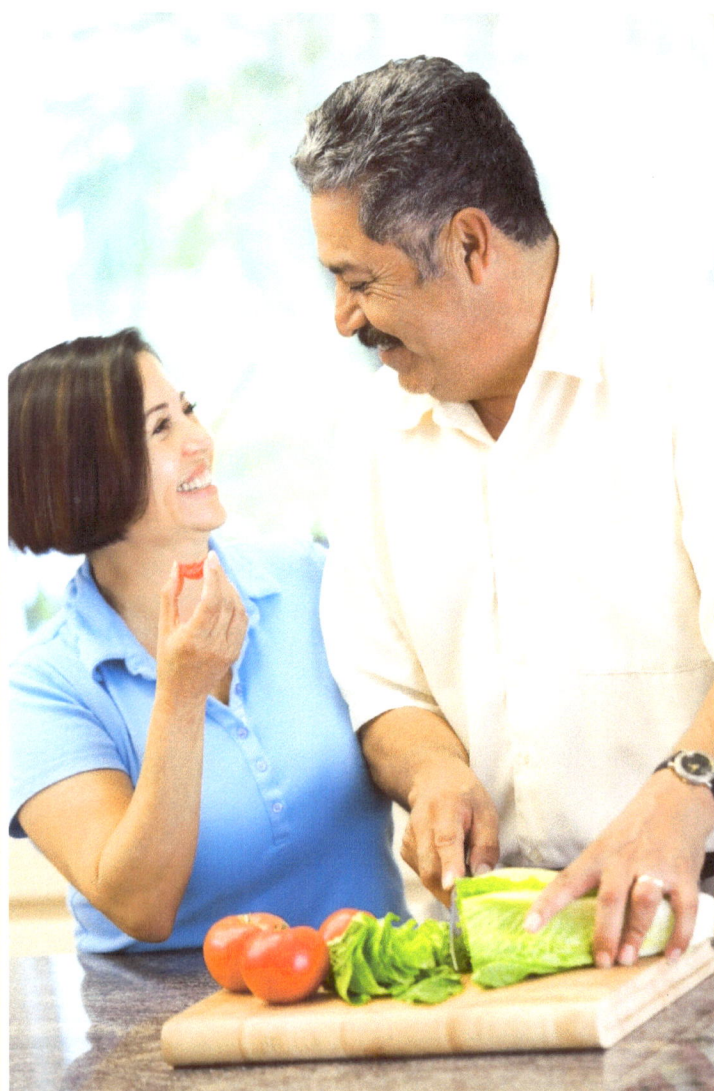

Follow these tips for reducing the fat (and increasing the fiber) in your diet:

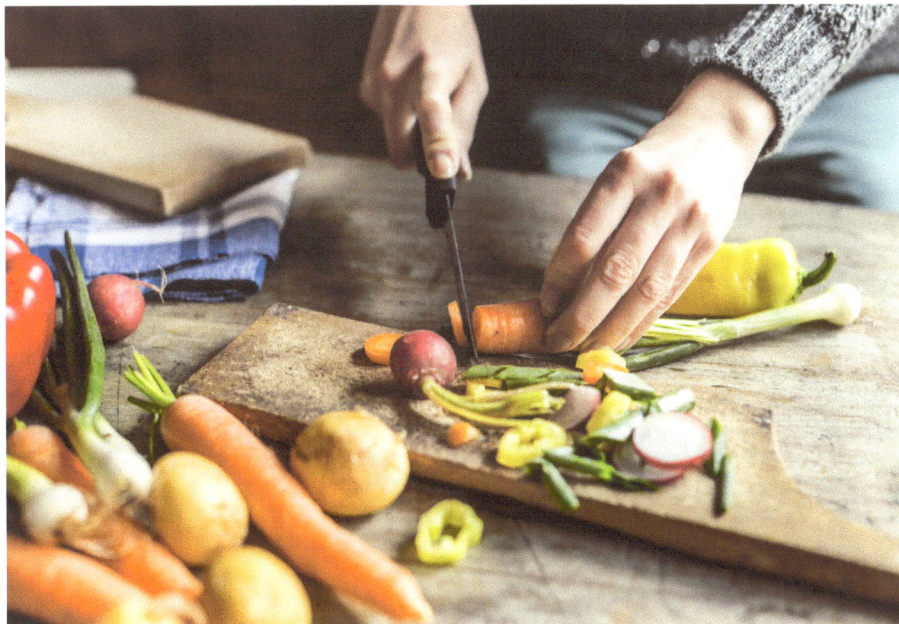

- bake, broil or poach meats

- remove the skin from chicken and turkey

- eat more fish and lean cuts of meat such as chicken or turkey

- use skim milk, 1% milk or evaporated skim milk instead of whole milk or 2% milk

- use low fat, low-sodium cheeses

- eat more fresh, frozen or canned fruit (in their own juices)

- eat more fresh, frozen or no salt added canned vegetables

- use less cream and cheese sauces (tomato sauces are OK)

- eat plain rice and pasta, English muffins, bagels, sandwich breads, soft tortillas

- eat whole grain cereals (cold or hot)

- use food labels to help you learn which foods are low in fat, cholesterol and sodium

- eat whole-grain breads and rice, dry peas and beans

Being physically inactive

Being inactive puts you at added risk for having CAD. **Regular** aerobic **exercise may help you reduce your risk** by:

- lowering bad cholesterol (LDL)

- raising good cholesterol (HDL)

- lowering blood pressure

- reducing excess weight

- toning and strengthening muscles, including the heart

- reducing stress

- lowering blood sugar

You should **check with your doctor before you begin or increase your physical activity.** Be careful if you have:

- high blood pressure

- pains or pressure in the chest or shoulder

- feel dizzy or faint

- get breathless after mild exertion

- have not been active

- are planning a vigorous workout program

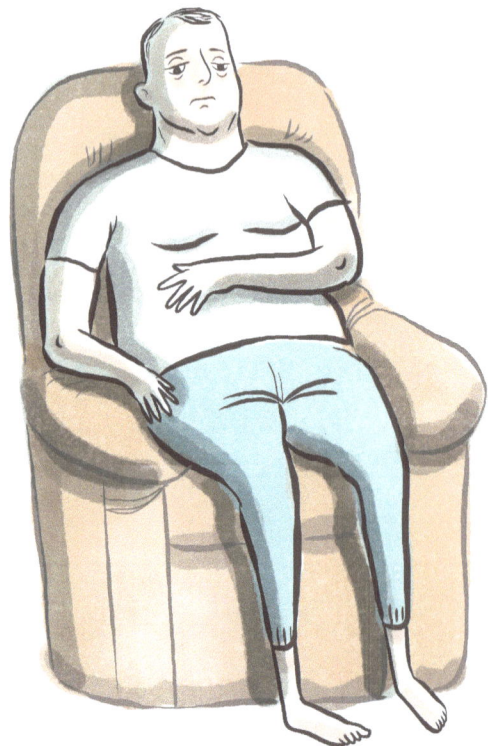

Regular, moderate exercise can help improve the way you look, feel and work. People who are not physically active are almost twice as likely to suffer from CAD as those who are active. Moderate aerobic exercise means doing the activity for 30 minutes a day most days of the week. Examples include:

- brisk walking

- jogging

- swimming

- bicycling

- playing tennis

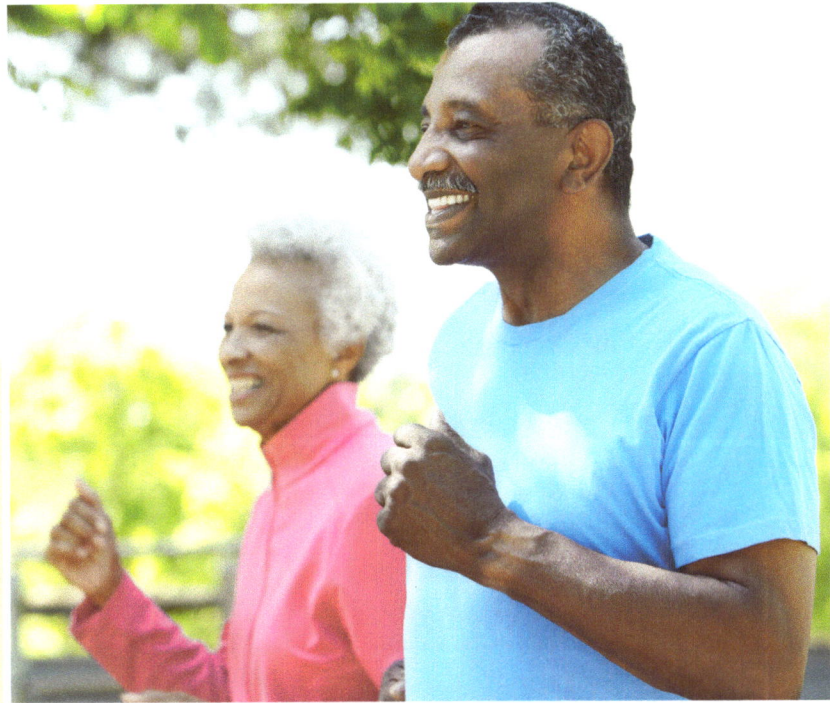

Even doing light to moderate activity for a few minutes most days may help you. Try:

- taking the stairs instead of the elevator or escalator

- doing some gardening

- doing housework

- dancing

Talk with your healthcare provider before you begin any exercise program. And always stop exercising at once if you have any pain, feel faint or light-headed or get really out of breath while exercising. Tell your doctor as soon as you can about this.

Unmanaged stress

Most of us are creatures of habit. We don't like change. Stress is caused by events that create change. These changes may be short lived (stuck in traffic) or long-term (death of a loved one). How well you handle change determines how stress affects you. People who have a problem handling change tend to have a lot of stress.

If you can accept that change has occurred and move on, then stress may not hurt you. (The traffic jam you're stuck in may make you late, but accept that there is not much you can do about it.) If, on the other hand, you dwell on these events and stay upset, it can bring on anxiety, chest pain or fast heartbeats.

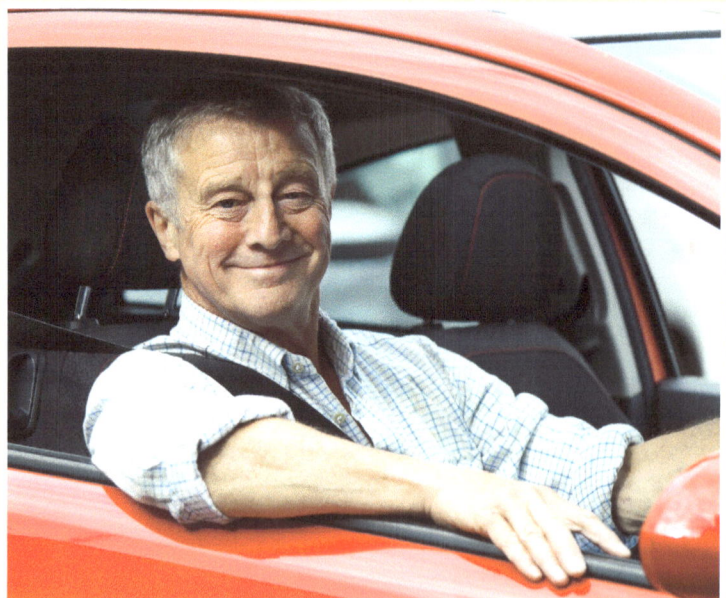

Although researchers cannot tell us why stress is a risk factor for CAD, they have noted that uncontrolled stress puts you at risk for the disease. Because stress varies from one person to another, stress levels are hard to judge. It may be that when you are under more stress, you do unhealthy things, like smoke, eat or drink too much.

Being relaxed and feeling good about yourself is good for your heart.

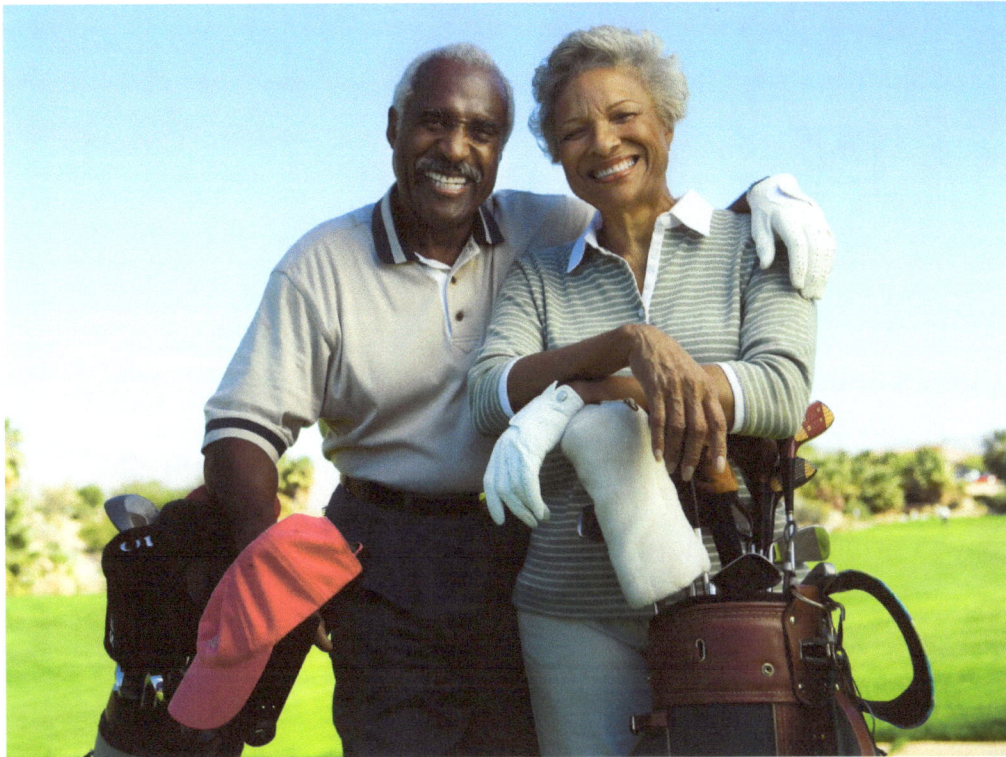

You will always have some stress in your life. You can't avoid it. Your goal is to learn to control it and not let it control you. Sometimes, this is easy to say and hard to do. See if these tips can help you:

- Try to be positive about your life.

- Learn to relax. You may need to use some relaxation techniques, like deep breathing exercises.

- Find time to play. Whatever you like to do—golf, tennis, sailing, hiking, reading poetry, etc.—make time to enjoy it.

- Eat healthy.

- Get physical. Exercise is a great stress reducer.

- Change your routine.

- Take a walk when you feel "uptight".

- Talk with a friend or loved one about how you feel.

- If you need to get organized and can't, get help.

- Laugh. Laughter can help reduce your stress.

Drinking too much alcohol

Drinking too much alcohol can raise blood pressure, cause irregular heartbeats and damage the heart muscle. It can also make high blood pressure harder to control.

If you don't drink, the best thing is not to start. If you do drink, limit how much you drink. Men should have no more than 2 drinks a day and women no more than 1 drink a day. A drink is defined as:

- 1½ oz of 80 proof whiskey or 1 oz of 100 proof whiskey

  or

- 5 oz of wine

  or

- 12 oz of beer
  (light or regular)

If you are trying to lose weight, keep in mind that alcohol contains calories—70 to 180 per drink (from the alcohol alone) depending on the drink.

Alcohol and many medicines do not mix. Check with your doctor or druggist about the medicines you take and ask about drinking alcohol while taking them.

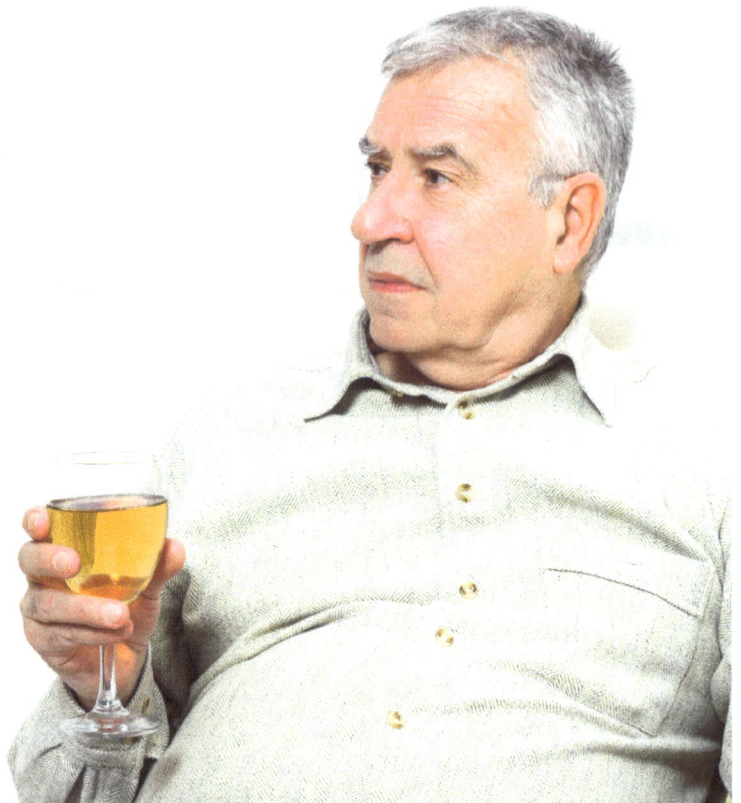

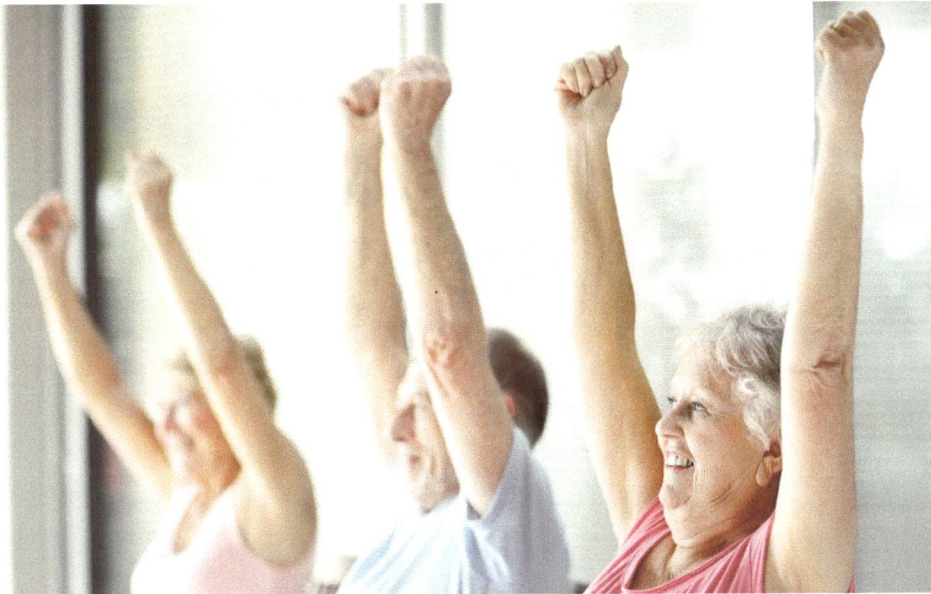

Now you know what to do!

Although a few factors cannot be changed, you now know ways to control the others. If you have any risks for CAD, here's what to do:

- make lifestyle changes—

    - lose weight, if you need to

    - don't use tobacco products

    - control your stress, learn to relax

    - limit your alcohol use

    - stay positive

    - follow a low-fat, low-cholesterol diet

    - do some aerobic exercise each day

- if you have diabetes, keep it well managed

- if you have high blood pressure, control it

What else can you do?

Work with your doctor to help reduce your risks for getting CAD. Keep him or her informed about what's going on in your life.

Know about any drug you take—what it's for and how much to take*. Make sure your doctor knows this too. This includes:

- all medicines—both prescribed and non-prescribed drugs (even aspirin)

- herbs

- vitamins

Some over-the-counter drugs and prescribed drugs can react badly when taken at the same time. The same is true for some herbal remedies and drugs.

If your doctor advises you to take a medicine to help reduce a risk factor, like high blood pressure, take it as prescribed. If you have any side effects while taking it, talk with your doctor.

You and your doctor should work together. Keep your doctor informed.

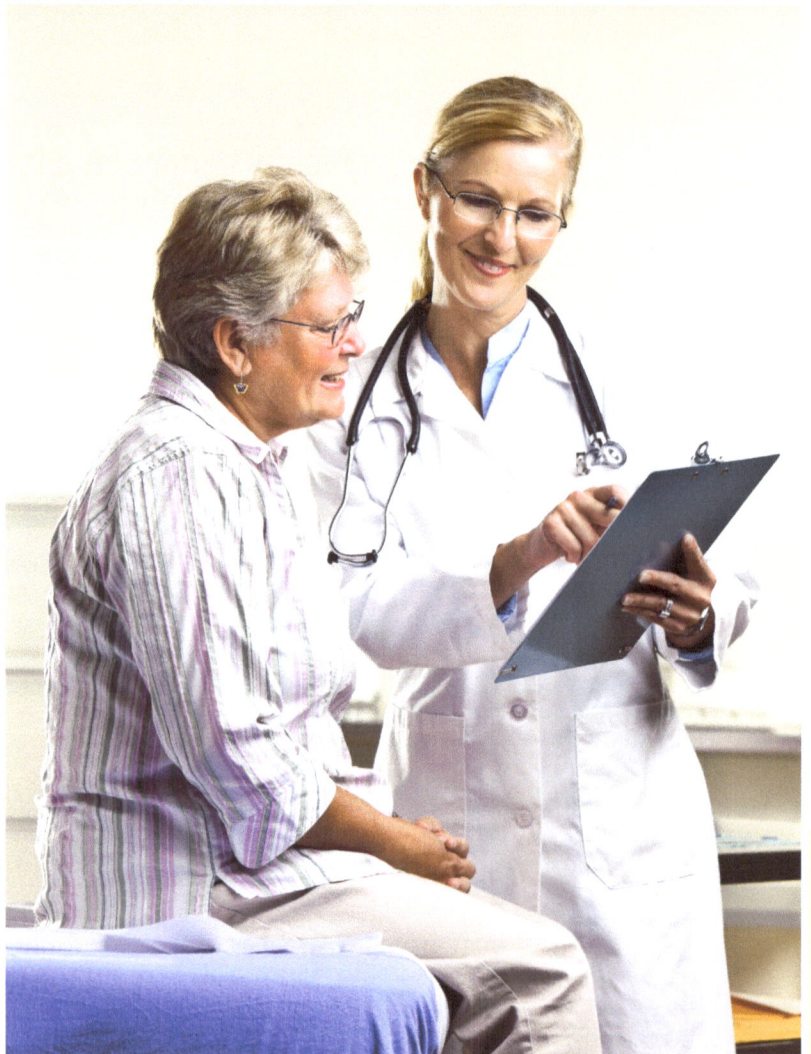

* Use the medicine chart on the next page.

Medicine chart

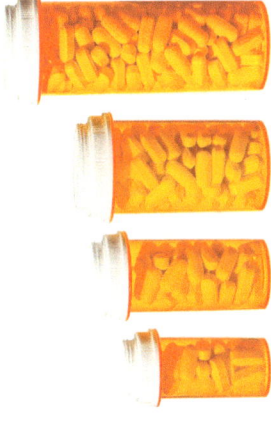

Ask your healthcare provider to help you fill in this medicine chart, and then keep it with you all the time. Make sure a loved one knows about it, too, in case of an emergency.

Name: _____

Dr.'s name: _____

Address: _____

Address: _____

Phone #: _____

Phone #: _____

Pharmacy: _____

Allergies I have:

Medicine name	What I take it for	How much I should take	Start date	How long to take it	When & how to take it	Side effects-Comments

Order this book from :

PRITCHETT & HULL ASSOCIATES, INC.
3440 OAKCLIFF RD NE STE 126
ATLANTA GA 30340-3006
or call toll free: 800-241-4925

Published and distributed by:
Pritchett & Hull Associates, Inc.
Printed in the U.S.A.

This book is written to help you
understand coronary artery disease.
It should not be used to replace any
of your doctor's advice or treatment.

www.ingramcontent.com/pod-product-compliance
Lightning Source LLC
Chambersburg PA
CBHW060854270326
41934CB00002B/131